# Introduction

Back pain is relatively common in the Un
as we age. It is estimated that 80% to 9
experience back pain within their lifetime.
for all physician visits and second most common complaint during a visit to a primary care physician. The exact cause of the pain varies depending on the mechanism of injury and structure injured, whether bone, muscle, ligament, or disc. The most common cause of pain is a muscle strain, although other causes include arthritis, disc herniation, ligament sprain, or fracture. The type and severity of symptoms will vary depending on the cause but will commonly lead to pain and loss of motion in the back region or lower extremity. If not treated appropriately, prolonged injury can lead to greater loss of mobility and function that can impact activities of daily living or one's ability to participate at work. This translates to an annual cost of 38 to 50 million dollars due to back pain alone. Plus, an estimated 25% to 50% of individuals will experience recurrent back pain episodes over the next year.

Fortunately, the most common causes of acute lower back pain are not serious and will improve over a relatively short period of time. Most symptoms may be treated over a several-week period with relative rest, medication, proper stretching, and improved posture. Subsequent symptoms may be prevented by continued stretching and strengthening of the back muscles. Prolonged or severe symptoms will require further treatment under the guidance of a physician to help prevent disability. The goal of this booklet is to describe the common causes of acute back pain relating to muscle strains and strategies for the prevention and treatment of such injuries.

## Structure (Anatomy) of the Back

The back is made up of bones, ligaments, and muscles that connect the torso to the lower body. It is designed to move the head and protect the spinal cord as it travels to the body. The various components of the neck are shown in Figures 1 to 7.

- The back or lumbar spine bones are called vertebrae, which are bones stacked one on top of another. There are five bones (L1–L5) plus the sacrum in the

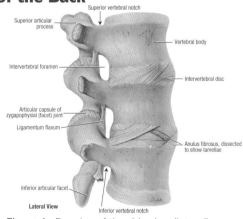

Figure 1. Drawing of the side view (lateral) lumbar spine.

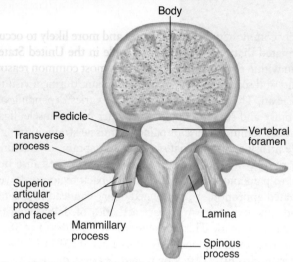

Body

Pedicle

Transverse
process

Superior
articular
process
and facet

Mammillary
process

Vertebral
foramen

Lamina

Spinous
process

*Figure 2.* Lumbar vertebra (L3), superior view. (From Tank PW, Gest TR. *Lippincott Williams & Wilkins Atlas of Anatomy*. Baltimore, MD: Lippincott Williams & Wilkins; 2009.)

back region. At the back of each vertebrae is an arch of bone that is designed to protect the spinal cord as it travels down the cervical spine to the rest of the body (Figs. 1 and 2).

- The lumbar spine nerves come off the spinal cord and travel through holes in the side of the bone (transverse foramen) before traveling to the hip and lower extremity (Fig. 3ab).
- In between the vertebrae are discs composed mostly of water and cartilage. The discs consist of an outer layer, called the annulus fibrosus, and an inner layer, called the nucleus pulposus. The outer layer is composed of alternating layers of cartilage (similar to your car tires) that provides strength when we twist and turn our neck. The inner layer is more like a jelly ball that helps lessen the forces to the neck when we bend and turn the head and neck region. As we age, the discs lose their water content and become stiffer. If a disc herniates, it will compress the spinal nerve near the intervertebral foramen leading to pain that radiates into the upper extremity (Fig. 4).
- Ligaments around the vertebrae act like guide wires that assist in movement of the back in multiple directions. The ligaments are broader in the front (anterior) of the spine than the back (posterior) of the spine near the spinal cord. The thinner posterior ligament covers less of the disc and is a potential area of weakness (Fig. 3ab).

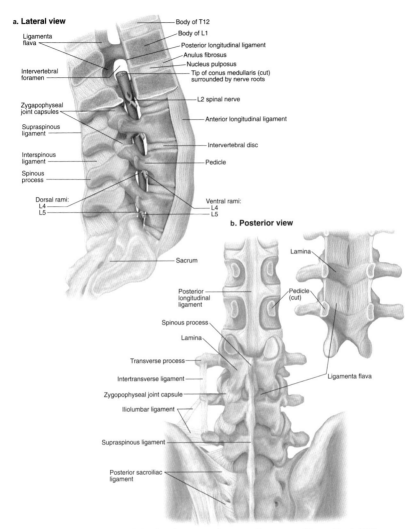

**a. Lateral view**

Ligamenta flava
Intervertebral foramen
Zygapophyseal joint capsules
Supraspinous ligament
Interspinous ligament
Spinous process
Dorsal rami:
L4
L5

Body of T12
Body of L1
Posterior longitudinal ligament
Anulus fibrosus
Nucleus pulposus
Tip of conus medullaris (cut) surrounded by nerve roots
L2 spinal nerve
Anterior longitudinal ligament
Intervertebral disc
Pedicle
Ventral rami:
L4
L5

Sacrum

**b. Posterior view**

Lamina
Posterior longitudinal ligament
Pedicle (cut)
Spinous process
Lamina
Transverse process
Intertransverse ligament
Zygapophyseal joint capsule
Iliolumbar ligament
Ligamenta flava
Supraspinous ligament
Posterior sacroiliac ligament

*Figure 3a,b.* Ligaments of the lumbar vertebrae and sacrum. (From Tank PW, Gest TR. *Lippincott Williams & Wilkins Atlas of Anatomy*. Baltimore, MD: Lippincott Williams & Wilkins; 2009.)

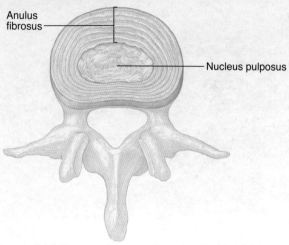

*Figure 4.* Intervertebral disc, superior view. (From Tank PW, Gest TR. *Lippincott Williams & Wilkins Atlas of Anatomy.* Baltimore, MD: Lippincott Williams & Wilkins; 2009.)

- Finally, there are multiple layers of muscles that provide additional support and assist with motion. Some muscles work over short distances to stabilize the various bones, whereas others work over longer distances to assist with rotation and bending of the spine. All of the structures must work in concert so you can turn your head sideways or up and down (Figs. 5 to 7).

## Imaging

Various imaging modalities allow us to look at the structures of the back when we are concerned about a serious injury. X-rays and CT scans are helpful in assessing bone alignment, arthritis, and fractures. In the normal standing position, the lumbar vertebrae are slightly curved in a reverse "C" shape as shown in Figure 8. With injury, the lumbar spine may straighten due to an underlying fracture or muscle spasm (Fig. 9). Excessive curvature or scoliosis of the lumbar spine may occur with other injuries or naturally to the spine (Fig. 10).

An MRI is useful for assessing disc herniations, the spinal cord, the ligaments, and the surrounding bony structures. Figure 11a shows a normal MRI of the spine from the side view (sagittal), whereas Figure 11b shows a lumbar disc herniation. Caution should be taken in looking at MRI as studies have shown that we develop abnormal images as we age, even though

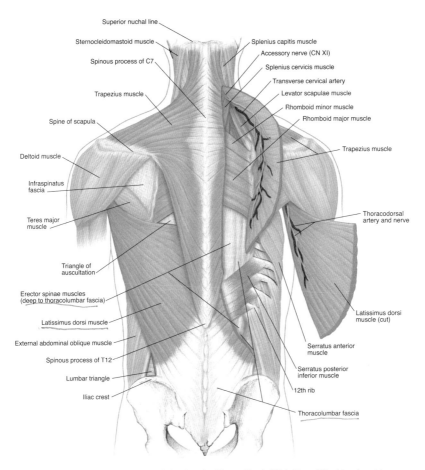

*Figure 5.* Superficial muscles of the back. (From Tank PW, Gest TR. *Lippincott Williams & Wilkins Atlas of Anatomy*. Baltimore, MD: Lippincott Williams & Wilkins; 2009.)

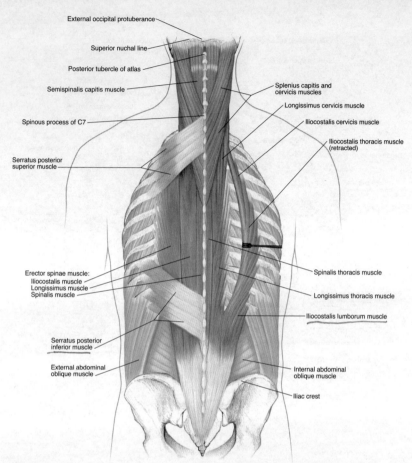

External occipital protuberance

Superior nuchal line

Posterior tubercle of atlas

Semispinalis capitis muscle

Spinous process of C7

Serratus posterior superior muscle

Erector spinae muscle:
Iliocostalis muscle
Longissimus muscle
Spinalis muscle

Serratus posterior inferior muscle

External abdominal oblique muscle

Splenius capitis and cervicis muscles

Longissimus cervicis muscle

Iliocostalis cervicis muscle

Iliocostalis thoracis muscle (retracted)

Spinalis thoracis muscle

Longissimus thoracis muscle

Iliocostalis lumborum muscle

Internal abdominal oblique muscle

Iliac crest

*Figure 6.* Deep back muscles, superficial dissection. (From Tank PW, Gest TR. *Lippincott Williams & Wilkins Atlas of Anatomy*. Baltimore, MD: Lippincott Williams & Wilkins; 2009.)

6

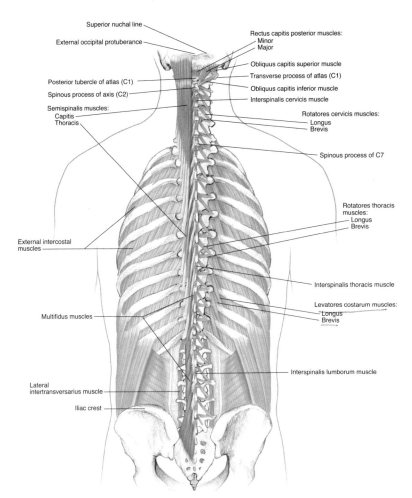

*Figure 7.* Deep back muscles, deeper dissection. (From Tank PW, Gest TR. *Lippincott Williams & Wilkins Atlas of Anatomy*. Baltimore, MD: Lippincott Williams & Wilkins; 2009.)

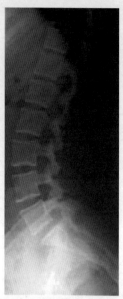

*Figure 8.* Lateral x-ray of the lumbar spine.

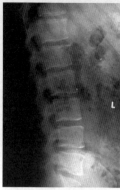

*Figure 9.* Lateral x-ray with straight lumbar spine.

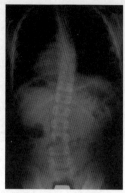

*Figure 10.* Lumbar spine x-ray with scoliosis.

we may not have symptoms. In studies of asymptomatic individuals, 38% exhibit disc bulges, 29% exhibit disc protrusions (slight herniation), 9.5% have disc extrusions (broken piece in the spinal cord), and more than 60% have at least one of these findings even though they have no pain. So speak with your doctor to better understand whether the MRI findings fit with your symptoms.

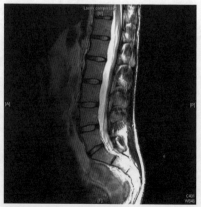

*Figure 11a.* Normal MRI of the lumbar spine (side view).

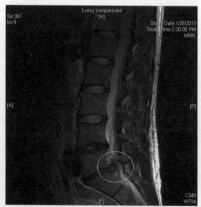

*Figure 11b.* Abnormal MRI of the lumbar spine showing a disc herniation.

# Common Injuries and Disease of the Back

Fortunately, the majority of injuries to the back are due to muscle ... Often, these injuries are due to nontraumatic mechanisms that may occur while performing an unfamiliar exercise or holding your back in an unnatural position. Conservative treatment as outlined in the following text can quickly alleviate most of the symptoms related to muscle strains. Any back pain that occurs due to trauma should be evaluated by a physician to assure there is no underlying fracture or injury to the spinal cord. In addition, back pain associated with tingling in the lower leg should be evaluated by a physician. In these cases, a thorough history, physical examination, and special imaging may be required to determine the cause of your symptoms. The following are common causes of back pain.

## Acute Muscle Strain

Muscle strains are the most common cause of acute lower back pain. These injuries typically occur during sudden, unexpected movement (i.e., quick rotation of the back while playing a sport/exercising) or slowly from poor posture during prolonged positions (i.e., bending over desk for hours, placing your computer too high/low, or sleeping in an uncomfortable position). The pain is described as achy to sharp in nature, involving the muscles around the back but not along the middle of the back. Often, the pain is worsened by bending forward or to the side, stretching the involved muscle. Although the pain may radiate to the gluteal region, it is not usually associated with tingling involving the lower leg. Coughing or sneezing does not typically worsen the pain. Pushing on the muscles of the lower back and stretching of the muscle will reproduce the pain. The majority (60% to 90%) of acute lower back muscle strains will usually resolve over a 6-week period with relative rest, avoidance of activity that exacerbates the symptoms, cold or heat packs, medication, and/or massage. A healthcare provider should evaluate symptoms lasting longer than the 6-week period. They may perform imaging to assess for other causes of neck pain and/or treat the symptoms with stronger pain medications, physical therapy, or injections.

## Disc Herniation

Back or lumbar disc herniations are less common—but more serious—injuries to the back. They are twice as likely to occur in males compared to females and often occur during 30 to 50 years of age. Other potential risk factors include lifting incorrectly, obesity, and smoking. The most common herniations occur at the L4–L5 and L5–S1 levels. A disc herniation occurs when the inner substance of the disc (nucleus pulposus) ruptures through the outer layer of the disc (annulus fibrosus), causing inflammation and compression of the nerves of the back. (Picture jelly coming out of a jelly donut [Fig. 12].) A disc herniation may occur when performing lifting activities or turning your head with the back flexed. Patients

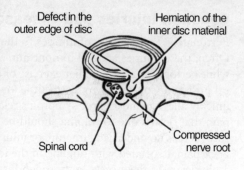

Figure 12. Lumbar disc herniation.

typically complain of sharp pain involving the region of the back with radiation of the pain to the lower leg. They may note tingling involving the thigh, leg, or foot in a specific area. The symptoms are worsened with bending forward and/or rotating to the same side. Coughing or sneezing will often make the symptoms worse. Anyone experiencing a potential disc herniation should seek a proper evaluation by a physician. Treatment can range from the use of medication, physical therapy, injections, and surgery, depending on the extent of the symptoms.

## Arthritis

Many of us get arthritis of the spine over time. However, not everyone has pain related to arthritis of the back. Arthritis occurs with increasing age as the cartilage wears away and the space between the bones narrows. Lumbar spine arthritis is quite uncommon in individuals younger than the age of 40 years. In the back, arthritis is associated with a loss in the height of the disc and overgrowth of the bone, which may narrow space for your nerves. Pain due to arthritis of the spine is gradual in onset, slowly occurring over weeks, months, or years. The pain is described as dull in nature and worsened with any movement of the back, especially extension. The pain may radiate toward the hip region but is not typically associated with tingling in the leg or foot unless the bony narrowing impinges a nerve. As the arthritis progresses, patients will describe pain with walking and improvement with leaning on a shopping cart while walking or sitting. Often, patients report back stiffness upon arising in the morning and lessening of the pain during the day with continued motion. Treatments include activity modification, pain medication, and exercise (stretching and strengthening). Arthritis that develops into significant narrowing of the spine may lead to loss of function of the extremities and/or balance issues. Therefore, it is important to seek an evaluation by your healthcare provider if you notice any of these symptoms.

## Preventive Measures

As noted before, a back strain may occur due to performing an unfamiliar exercise or holding the back in an unnatural position. Common positions or deficits that can lead to subsequent back strain include

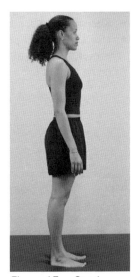

*Figure 13a.* Good posture.

1. Poor abdominal and lumbar spine muscle strength: (Fig. 13b) Proper strength of these muscles is essential to maintaining proper posture (Fig. 13a) and preventing subsequent injury. Strength of these "core" muscles will protect the spine when it is in an unusual or awkward position.
2. Bending forward while lifting a heavy object off the ground may place an unusual stress on the back. People usually experience a disc herniation while bending forward with rotation.
3. Holding the back rotated or twisted for a prolonged period of time.

Patients may find themselves in any of these positions during common daily activities. Any task in which the back is flexed and bent over a work—such as working at a desk or on a computer, or lifting a heavy object—may cause strain to the back muscles. Even resting can cause back strain if it is done in an improper position and too often. Finally, other associated factors contributing to possible back pain include smoking, depression, anxiety, poor job satisfaction, and lack of aerobic conditioning.

Figures 14 through 31 illustrate unnatural body positions that are common causes of back strains during everyday activities. In addition, the figures note the proper positions to help prevent such injury. If your back pain impacts your ability

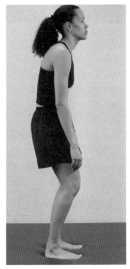

*Figure 13b.* Poor spine posture.

to perform your job, you should consider a "work-site evaluation" to assure the proper placement of your work equipment, such as your computer, to help prevent subsequent injury.

Tips:
- Keep your back straight while sitting in a chair (Figs. 14 and 15).
- Use a chair with proper support of the back, shoulders, and arms to prevent your head from being thrust forward and your back from being curved for a prolonged period of time (Figs. 16 and 17).

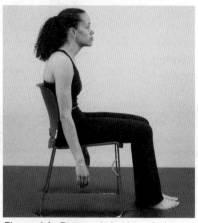

*Figure 14*. Person sitting in a chair, slouched forward.

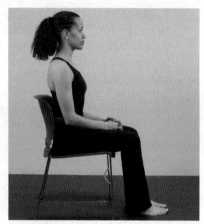

*Figure 15*. Person sitting in a chair with correct posture.

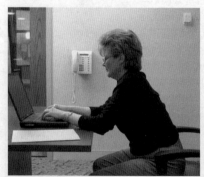

*Figure 16*. Person working on a desk, leaning forward.

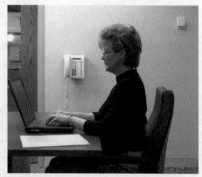

*Figure 17*. Person working on a desk with proper posture and chair support.

- Make sure your chair is the right height, neither too low nor too high. Sit straight and avoid having to twist or stretch forward while working, eating, and so forth (Figs. 18 and 19).

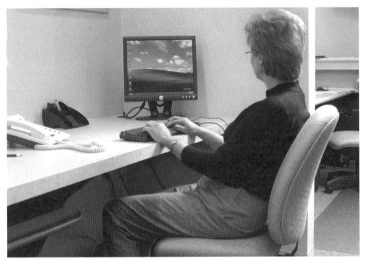

*Figure 18.* Person at the desk slouching and rotated while typing on a computer.

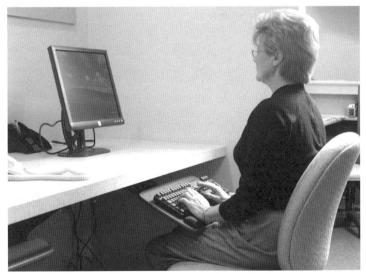

*Figure 19.* Person with proper alignment of work site to type on a computer.

- Make sure your car seat is adjusted properly. If it is too far forward, you will need to stretch your back forward to see (Figs. 20 and 21).

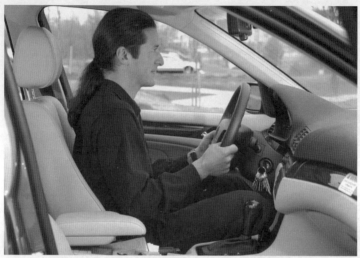

*Figure 20.* Person driving in car with incorrect posture.

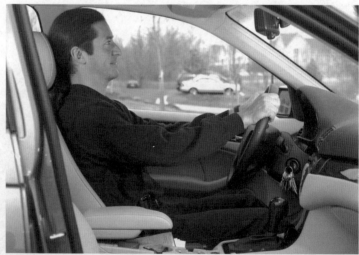

*Figure 21.* Person driving in car with correct posture.

- Bend at the knees and not the waist to reach for drawers that are lower to the ground (Figs. 22 and 23).

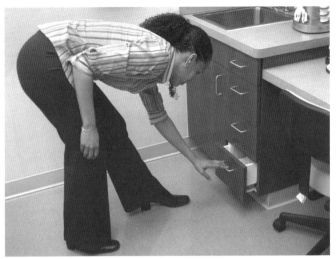

*Figure 22.* Person bending to open drawer with poor posture.

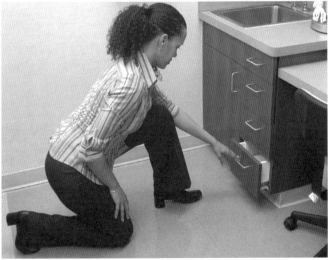

*Figure 23.* Person bending to open drawer with correct posture.

- While reading in bed, sit with proper lower back support (Figs. 24 and 25).

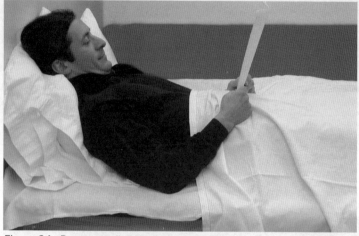

*Figure 24.* Person reading in a bed, slouching.

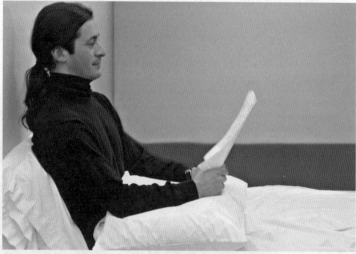

*Figure 25.* Person sitting in bed with proper posture.

- Avoid bending at the waist when sweeping, raking, or shoveling (Figs. 26 and 27).

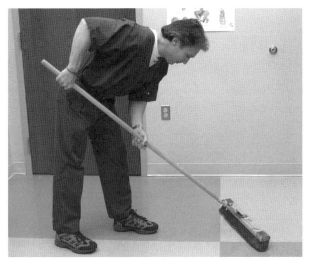

*Figure 26.* Person sweeping with poor posture.

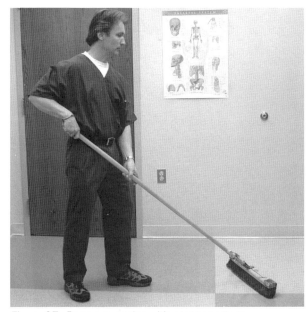

*Figure 27.* Person sweeping with proper posture.

- Lift objects by bending your knees, not your waist. Remember to breathe normally as you lift the object (Figs. 28 and 29).

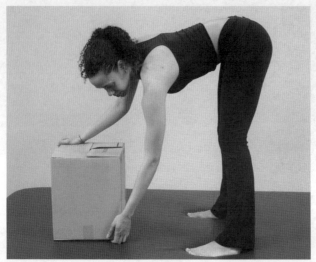

*Figure 28.* Bending forward with incorrect posture.

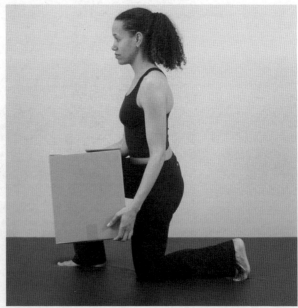

*Figure 29.* Lifting by squatting down, perhaps one leg behind.

- Hold boxes close to the body to prevent excessive strain on the back muscles (Figs. 30 and 31).

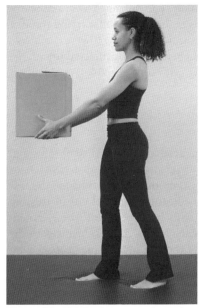

*Figure 30.* Holding box away from the body.

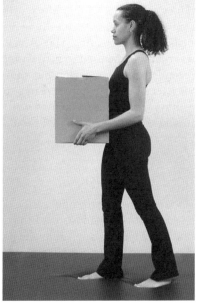

*Figure 31.* Holding box near body.

# Treatment Options

Proper treatment of any back injury requires supervision by a physician, especially when there is trauma to the back, prolonged pain, or associated tingling involving the lower leg. Fortunately, patients have a variety of options to treat back pain symptoms. Patients should consider trying some of these basic options prior to seeking medical attention. However, patients should be sure to discuss with the physician any treatments and obtain the physician's approval before progressing with any exercises, especially if they worsen back pain.

## Medication

A variety of medications may be used to relieve back pain symptoms and improve recovery. The most common medications are called NSAIDs or nonsteroidal anti-inflammatory drugs. Common NSAIDs include ibuprofen, naproxen, or meloxicam. These medications are helpful in treating the pain and inflammation associated with back pain. However, potential side effects include acid reflux, stomach ulcers, and problems with the kidneys. Patients should always discuss the use of any medication with a physician to ensure that there are no issues preventing the use of such medications in treating pain. Acetaminophen is another common medication that may be used to help with pain relief. It has fewer side effects and is gentler on the stomach but should be used cautiously in anyone who has liver disease. Topical creams such as BenGay or IcyHot may provide symptomatic relief of pain as well. Other medications such as narcotics, muscle relaxers, or tramadol should only be used under the supervision of a physician.

## Modalities and Bracing

Modalities include the application of such interventions as ice, heat, electrical stimulation, or ultrasound to the muscles of the back. Several of these modalities may be applied by the patient. Others require a licensed professional trained in its proper use.

- *Ice*: After acute injury, you should use ice for any muscle pain to reduce pain and swelling. Ice is the preferred modality to be used intermittently for the first 48 hours following an injury. Although, it may be used longer if you find it is helping your symptoms. Cold packs, frozen vegetable packs, or ice bags can be used. Ice packs should be wrapped in a cloth or towel so that they are not placed directly on the skin. Direct application to skin can be uncomfortable and cause damage to skin. Ice packs are most helpful if used several times a day for approximately 10 to 15 minutes.

- *Heat*: Heat helps relieve pain and promotes circulation and muscle relaxation. Heating packs, electric heating pads, or moist-heated towels can be used. Moist heat, as applied through a hot pack or warm towel, should be applied to the involved area to help relax your muscles prior to performing gentle stretching exercises. Heat should be used cautiously in the first 48 hours because it may increase the amount of inflammation and swelling. Heat packs should be wrapped in a cloth or towel so that they are not placed directly on the skin. Direct application to skin can be uncomfortable and burn the skin.
- *Ultrasound*: This modality utilizes heat and ultrasound waves to treat your muscle pain. Ultrasound treatment should only be applied by a professional trained in its proper use.
- *Electrical stimulation*: Electrical stimulation as applied through E-Stim or a TENS unit can assist with the reduction of pain. Similar to the use of ultrasound, the treatment should only be applied by a professional trained in its proper use.
- *Massage*: Gentle massage, consisting of kneading or stroking of the back muscles, can help alleviate some pain. However, massage is most effective when administered by a licensed professional massage therapist.
- *Back brace*: At times, some physicians will prescribe a back brace to relieve some of the stress to the muscles of your back. However, you should not use the back brace for more than a few days because prolonged use will lead to deconditioning of the back muscles and worsening pain.

## Physical Therapy

For more severe pain, your physician may prescribe physical therapy to treat your back pain symptoms depending on the cause of your pain. Physical therapists will utilize a variety of the modalities listed earlier to decrease your pain and increase your back's range of motion. You will then progress to a series of back stretching and strengthening exercises. These exercises are listed in the following text and should be incorporated into a home exercise program. It is extremely important to perform your exercises on a daily basis to assist in recovery and prevent deconditioning of the muscles of the neck.

Injection techniques may include interventions such as acupuncture, trigger point injections, or injections into the spine. Chronic muscle pains may respond to acupuncture or trigger point injections. In theory, they assist in relaxing the muscle by inhibiting an area of spasm. Interventional spinal procedures may include injections to the spinal nerves (epidural or transforaminal) if there is a disc herniation or joints (facets) if the pain is due to arthritis. A specially trained practitioner should only perform these procedures.

## Exercises

The following series of exercises is specifically designed to stretch and strengthen the muscles in your back. If you are recovering from a back strain or have chronic stiffness, you should start the exercises slowly and gradually build up your strength and endurance until you can perform them several times per day. Mild increased soreness or stiffness may occur the day after performing these exercises. However, prolonged or worsening pain should lead to an evaluation by your physician. You should discuss your exercise program with your doctor before you begin and keep your doctor informed of your progress and any problems or questions. These exercises should be incorporated into a general exercise program that includes aerobic conditioning, such as walking, running, or cycling.

### Stretching

The following stretches are designed to help increase your back's range of motion. You should hold each stretch for 20 to 30 seconds and repeat each stretch two to three times, at least once a day. You should stretch the muscle until you feel a slight pull, but no further.

**Exercise 1:** <u>Lumbar spine stretch:</u> knees to chest. Lie flat on your back with your knees slightly bent. Very slowly bring your right knee toward your chest, while keeping your left knee bent with your left foot on the floor. You may grab the back of your right leg with your hands to further stretch the lower back. Hold the position for 20 seconds (Fig. 32). Slowly return to the starting position and repeat on the other side.

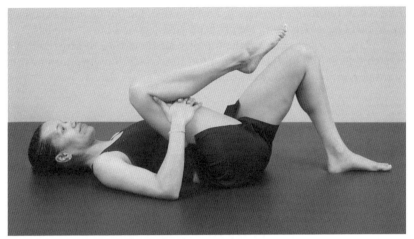

*Figure 32.* Lumbar stretch—supine, knees to chest.

**Exercise 2:** <u>Lumbar spine stretch:</u> sitting. Sit in a firm, sturdy chair. Hold your arms loosely by your sides. Lower your head toward your knees, bending at the waist. Hold the position for 20 seconds (Fig. 33). Slowly return to your starting position.

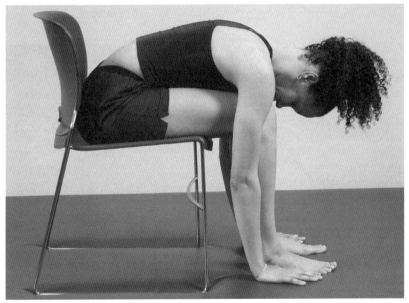

*Figure 33.* Lumbar stretch, sitting.

**Exercise 3:** <u>Lumbar spine stretch:</u> knees to side. Lie flat on your back with your knees bent (Fig. 34a). Slowly bend your legs and hips to the left. You may place your left hand on the top of your right knee to assist with the stretch (Fig 34b). Hold the position for 20 seconds. Slowly return to your starting position. Repeat to the opposite side.

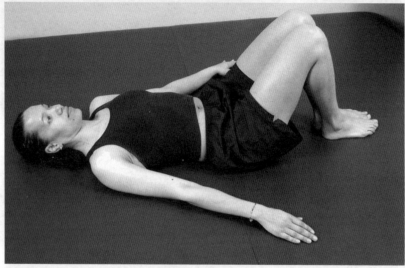

*Figure 34a.* Lumbar stretch—supine, knees to side start position.

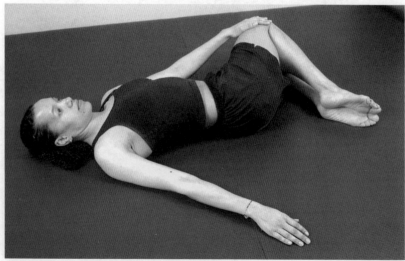

*Figure 34b.* Lumbar stretch—supine, knees to side exercise.

**Exercise 4:** <u>Lumbar spine stretch:</u> prone. Support yourself on your hands and knees (Fig. 35a). Gently round your back like a cat (Fig. 35b), hold for 20 seconds, and return to your starting position.

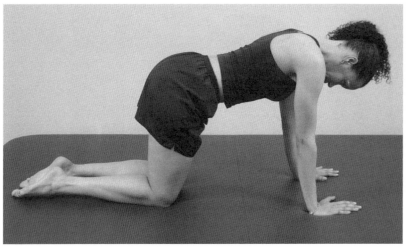

*Figure 35a.* Cat lumbar stretch start position.

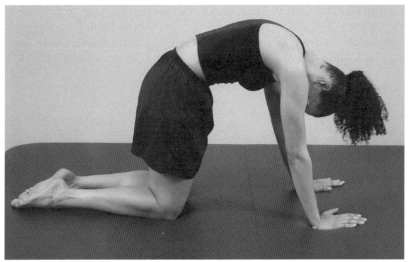

*Figure 35b.* Cat lumbar stretch exercise.

**Exercise 5:** <u>Hamstring stretch:</u> sitting. Sit on the floor with your legs closed in front of you. Gently lean forward with your chest, keeping your lower back straight until you feel a pull in the hamstring region (Fig. 36). Keep your knees straight.

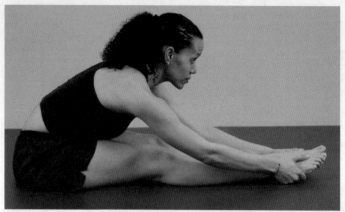

*Figure 36.* Hamstring stretch, sitting.

**Exercise 6:** <u>Hip flexor stretch:</u> (Caution: Perform this exercise on a mat to minimize any knee discomfort.) Start with your weight on your right knee and left foot. Gently lean forward with your left knee to produce a stretch in the front of the right hip (Fig. 37). Make sure to keep your left knee directly above your ankle, not forward over your toes. Return to your starting position and repeat on the other side.

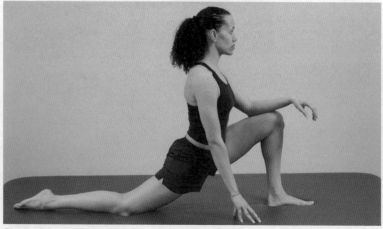

*Figure 37.* Hip flexor stretch.

**Exercise 7:** <u>Quadriceps stretch:</u> Start by standing with both feet together and your hands by your sides. While standing on your left leg, grab your right foot on the opposite leg with your right hand and pull the foot toward the buttock region until you feel a pull in your thigh (Fig. 38a). Remember to keep your pelvis level and your foot toward the middle of the buttock region (Fig. 38b shows incorrect position). Return to your starting position and repeat on the other side. If this is too difficult, you may perform the same maneuver while lying on your stomach (Fig. 38c).

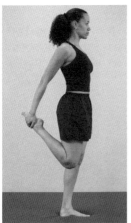 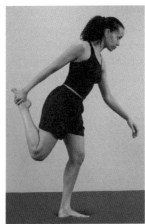

*Figure 38a.* CORRECT.     *Figure 38b.* INCORRECT.

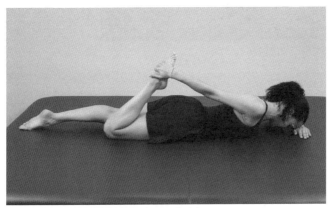

*Figure 38c.* CORRECT. Quad stretch, lying.

## Strengthening

After your pain has decreased and your range of motion has improved, you may gradually start your strengthening exercise program. These back exercises are designed to increase your overall strength and stamina. You should hold each position for approximately 3 to 5 seconds and relax. Repeat each exercise three to five times as tolerated. Be sure to breathe properly throughout the exercises. For individuals under the guidance of a physical therapist or personal trainer, more complex strengthening exercises will be combined with functional exercises to promote a safe and speedy return to sporting activity.

**Exercise 1:** <u>Pelvic tilts.</u> Lie on your back with your knees bent (Fig. 39a). Gently pull your navel toward the floor as your pelvis slowly rotates up from the bottom (Fig. 39b). Hold the position for 5 seconds and return to the starting position. Repeat three to five times.

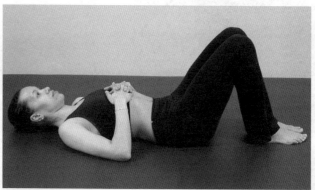

*Figure 39a.* Pelvic tilts start position.

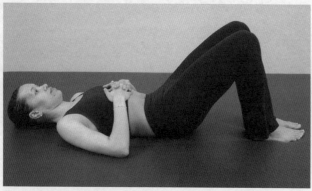

*Figure 39b.* Pelvic tilts exercise.

**Exercise 2:** <u>Dead bug.</u> Lie on your back with your legs flat on the ground and your left arm over your head (Fig. 40a). Gently lift your right leg and left arm several inches off the floor (Fig. 40b). Hold the position for 5 seconds and return to the starting position. Repeat three to five times and on the opposite side.

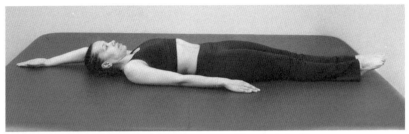

*Figure 40a.* Supine, dead bug opposite arm and leg start position.

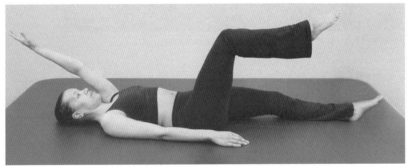

*Figure 40b.* Supine, dead bug opposite arm and leg exercise.

**Exercise 3:** <u>Superman.</u> Start on your hands and knees with a flat back (Fig. 41a). Gently lift your right leg and left arm until they are in line with your spine (Fig. 41b). Hold the position for 5 seconds and return to the starting position. Repeat on the opposite side.

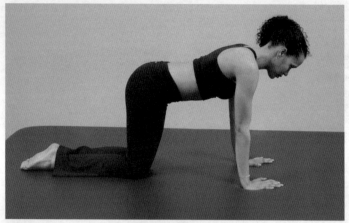

*Figure 41a.* Prone, opposite arm and leg start position.

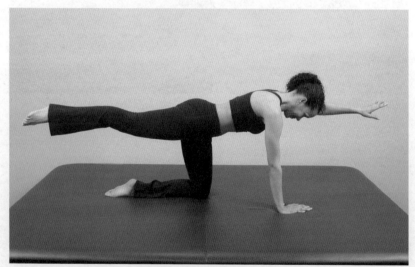

*Figure 41b.* Prone, opposite arm and leg exercise.

**Exercise 4:** <u>Abdominal exercises.</u> Lie on your back with your knees bent and hands behind your head or crossed on your chest (Fig. 42a). Gently lift your head and upper torso several inches off the floor by tightening your abdominal muscles (Fig. 42b). Hold the position for 5 seconds and return to the starting position.

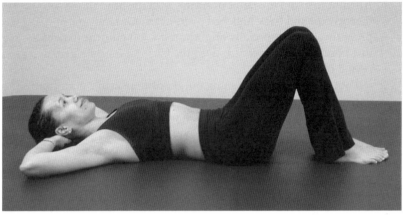

*Figure 42a.* Abdominal exercise start position.

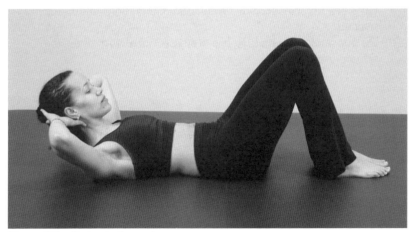

*Figure 42b.* Abdominal exercise.

# Summary

1. Back pain is often due to muscle strains, which can be treated by proper rest, activity modification, medication, and exercises to improve posture. Severe back pain or stiffness that does not respond to the earlier interventions could indicate a more serious problem that requires medical attention.
2. Attempt to avoid the habit of sitting with the head thrust too far forward and back hunched over. Learn to stand and sit properly. This is especially important if a job puts the patient in a position that causes strain to the back for a prolonged period of time.
3. Do not slump or slouch in unnatural positions while performing daily activities.
4. The patient should be sure to get enough rest. Stress and tiredness can contribute to back pain symptoms.
5. Exercise to stretch and strengthen the muscles in the back. The patient should perform these exercises several times per week to maintain proper flexibility and strength.
6. The patient should incorporate back exercises into a generalized exercise program including aerobic conditioning.
7. Maintain a healthy weight, as obesity may place increased pressure on the structures of your spine.
8. Eat a healthy, balanced diet to maintain good bone and muscle structure.
9. Do not smoke, as smoking has been associated with degeneration of discs.

RRS1806